PROLAPSE AND WOMEN:

Symptoms, Prevention, and Treatment

Kelly Brown

Table of Contents

CHAPTER ONE

Introduction

Millions of women throughout the globe suffer with pelvic organ prolapse, a common but sometimes misunderstood medical ailment. A woman's quality of life and general wellbeing may be greatly affected by this illness, which is defined by the descent or bulging of pelvic organs such as the bladder, uterus, or rectum into the vaginal canal. Prolapse in women is a subject of great significance to the field of women's health and warrants thorough investigation and comprehension.

The female pelvis is a wonder of anatomical intricacy, supporting the uterus, bladder, and rectum, among other important organs. The pelvic floor, a network of muscles, ligaments, and connective tissues, holds these organs firmly in place. The disconcerting incidence of pelvic organ prolapse might result from a weakening or breakdown of this complex network of support.

Women have prolapse for a variety of reasons, often a combination of causes. For example, pregnancy and childbirth have a big role because they put a lot of pressure on the pelvic floor, which might compromise its structural integrity. Pelvic organ prolapse may also be brought on by other elements including age, hormonal changes, persistent constipation, and obesity.

The degree of prolapse symptoms may vary, and they cover a broad spectrum of pain and misery. Women who have prolapse may feel pressure in the pelvis, "something coming down" in the vagina, incontinence, trouble going to the bathroom, and even discomfort when having sex. The physical, emotional, and social well-being of a woman may be significantly impacted by these symptoms, which often result in shame, worry, and a worse quality of life.

There are efficient care and treatment options for pelvic organ prolapse, ranging from changes in lifestyle and pelvic floor exercises to surgical procedures. However, for women to make wise choices regarding their health, they must be aware of the illness, its risk factors, and the available treatment options.

We shall go more into the complexities of prolapse in women in this investigation. We will cover its different manifestations, underlying causes, and risk factors, as well as the potential medical and psychological effects it may have on people who encounter it. We will also go through the many diagnostic procedures and treatment choices, giving women the information they need to seek the right medical attention and reclaim their lives.

We want to be a useful resource for persons suffering from this problem, their loved ones, and healthcare professionals alike with our thorough investigation of prolapse in women. Understanding the complexity of pelvic organ prolapse can help us all work together to improve the health and wellbeing of women. Knowledge is a powerful weapon.

CHAPTER TWO:

Overview of Women's Prolapse

Prolapse is a medical disorder that predominantly affects women and causes the pelvic area's organs to move out of their normal places or descend. Vital organs including the uterus, bladder, rectum, and vaginal walls are all located in the pelvic region and are all susceptible to prolapse. This syndrome develops when the pelvic muscles and supporting tissues deteriorate or are injured, enabling the organs to move below.

Women may encounter a number of prolapse kinds, including:

Uterine Prolapse: The uterus may prolapse and enter the vaginal canal. Age, childbearing, and weakening of the pelvic floor muscles are a few causes of this.

Bladder Prolapse (Cystocele): When the vagina's front wall becomes weak, the bladder may protrude into the vaginal area. A urinary condition may result from this.

Rectal prolapse: When the rectum protrudes through the anus, it causes pain and problems with bowel movements. It may be connected to straining or ongoing constipation.

Following a hysterectomy, a woman may have vaginal vault prolapse, which includes the top section of the vagina descending into the vaginal canal.

Numerous pregnancies, delivery, age and hormonal changes, obesity, persistent constipation or straining during bowel movements, and a hereditary tendency to weak connective tissues are some of the reasons for prolapse, but they might vary.

Pelvic pressure or heaviness, a sense of something protruding into or out of the vagina, urine incontinence, problems going to the bathroom, and pain during sexual activity are all signs of prolapse.

Depending on the degree and kind of prolapse, treatment options for it vary from dietary changes and pelvic floor exercises (like Kegel exercises) to the use of pessaries (vaginal devices) and surgical treatments. A woman's quality of life may be considerably enhanced and further issues can be avoided with early identification and treatment.

Prolapse is a disorder that may have a significant negative effect on a woman's physical and mental health, but many women can successfully manage and reduce its symptoms with the right medical treatment and assistance, allowing them to enjoy happy, productive lives. It is crucial to see a healthcare provider for a precise diagnosis and individualized treatment plan if you think you may have prolapse or are exhibiting symptoms that are connected to it.

Prolapse types

Abdominal Prolapse:

When the uterus dips or sags into the vaginal canal, uterine prolapse develops. It belongs to the most prevalent categories of prolapse.

The muscles and ligaments of the pelvic floor are frequently compromised as a consequence of childbirth, repeated pregnancies, obesity, and age.

Women who have uterine prolapse may suffer pelvic pressure, lower back pain, urine incontinence, and a feeling that something is pushing into their vagina.

Cystocele, or bladder prolapse:

The protrusion of the bladder into the front (front) vaginal wall is known as a cystocele. The bladder may protrude into the vaginal canal as a result.

Causes: Primary reasons include anterior vaginal wall and pelvic floor thinning, which are often linked to childbearing and age.

Urinary urgency, repeated UTIs, inability to fully empty the bladder, and a sensation of pressure or fullness in the pelvic region are all typical symptoms.

Rectal Prolapse: Definition: Rectal prolapse occurs when the rectum protrudes through the anus, causing a reddish mass to appear outside the body.

Rectal prolapse may have a variety of causes, including heredity, weak pelvic floor muscles, chronic constipation, and straining during bowel movements.

Symptoms: People who have rectal prolapse may have trouble managing their bowel movements, fecal incontinence, and discomfort or pain while going to the bathroom.

Vaginal Vault Prolapse: Definition: Women who have had hysterectomy (the removal of the uterus) are more likely to have this form of prolapse. The vaginal canal is reached via the upper portion of the vagina.

Vaginal vault prolapse may be brought on by the weakening of the tissues that support the vagina following a hysterectomy.

Symptoms: Women may feel as if their vaginas are swelling, as well as pelvic pressure, pain, and sexual problems.

An area of the small intestine protrudes into the upper vaginal wall in an enterocele, a less frequent kind of prolapse.

Causes: Weaker pelvic floor muscles and ligaments are the main causes, similar to other prolapses.

Symptoms: Pelvic pressure, discomfort, and sometimes pain or discomfort during sexual activity are possible symptoms.

Perineal Prolapse (Perineocele): The perineum, or the region between the vaginal entrance and the anus, descends in perineal prolapse. It could cause a bulge or sagging in this area.

Perineal prolapse may be caused by weakening of the pelvic floor and the tissues that support the perineum.

Symptoms: There may be an obvious protrusion, pressure or pain in the perineal region, and problems going to the bathroom.

Causes and Prolapse Risk Factors

There are many reasons and risk factors that might contribute to prolapse in females. For treatment and prevention, it is crucial to comprehend these elements. The following list includes prolapse's risk factors and causes:

1. Childbirth: Childbirth, especially vaginal births, is one of the main causes of pelvic organ prolapse. During labor and delivery, the muscles and connective tissues of the pelvic floor are stretched and perhaps injured, weakening the support systems for the pelvic organs and raising the risk of prolapse.

2. Aging: As women age, the normal aging process may result in a loss of suppleness and muscular tone in the tissues surrounding the pelvic floor. This age-related deterioration may be a factor in prolapse.

3. Hormonal Changes: Prolapse is more probable as a result of hormonal changes, notably the drop in estrogen that occurs after menopause, which may cause tissue elasticity and strength to diminish in the pelvic region.

4. Obesity: Carrying around extra pounds puts additional strain on the tissues and muscles of the pelvic floor, which over time may weaken and raise the risk of prolapse.

5. Chronic constipation and straining: Prolapse may be exacerbated by repeated straining during bowel movements, which is often linked to chronic constipation.

6. hereditary Predisposition: Prolapse may be more likely in certain women due to a hereditary predisposition to structural difficulties in the pelvic area or weaker connective tissues.

7. several Pregnancies: Due to the accumulated stress on the pelvic floor, women who have had several pregnancies and births may be more susceptible to prolapse.

8. Heavy Lifting: Lifting heavy things on a regular basis may put pressure on the pelvic floor and raise the risk of prolapse, particularly if it is done incorrectly and with poor body mechanics.

9. Chronic Coughing: Irregular coughing, chronic bronchitis, and asthma may all increase intra-abdominal pressure, which puts strain on the pelvic floor and promotes prolapse.

10. Pelvic Surgery: Past pelvic operations, particularly hysterectomy (removal of the uterus), may change the pelvic anatomy and impair support systems, which may result in prolapse.

11. Connective Tissue Disorders: Prolapse is more likely to occur if a person has a connective tissue condition like Ehlers-Danlos syndrome or Marfan syndrome, which may damage the strength and integrity of pelvic tissues.

12. Ethnicity and Genetic Factors: According to certain research, differences in pelvic anatomy and genetic predispositions may make some ethnic groups more susceptible to prolapse.

It's crucial to remember that not all women with these risk factors will have prolapse, and not every instance of prolapse has a definite, observable cause. Maintaining a healthy weight, strengthening the pelvic floor with exercises like Kegels, and getting medical help if prolapse symptoms develop are common components of prevention and treatment techniques. Early management may reduce symptoms and enhance the afflicted person's overall quality of life. For individualized advice and treatment, speak with a healthcare professional if you believe you may have prolapse or are at risk.

CHAPTER THREE:

Women's Prolapse Symptoms

Women who have prolapse may suffer a variety of symptoms, and the particular symptoms they encounter may depend on the kind and degree of the prolapse. Here are some typical signs and symptoms of various prolapse types:

1. Pelvic Pressure: A persistent feeling of fullness, pressure, or heaviness in the pelvic area is a common prolapse symptom. The severity of this sensation may change during the day, even becoming worse.

2. Bulging Sensation: Many prolapse sufferers report feeling a lump or bulge in the vaginal or rectal region, which may

enlarge when they stand, cough, or exert themselves.

Urinary Symptoms: 3.

Urinary Incontinence: Prolapse may cause stress urinary incontinence, which results in urine leaking when you laugh, sneeze, or exert yourself physically.

Frequency and Urgency: Common symptoms include a sudden, intense need to pee and a rise in urine frequency.

Bladder Emptying Difficulties: Some prolapsed women may have trouble fully emptying their bladders.

4. Constipation: Prolapse may make it harder to pass stools or cause persistent constipation.

Fecal Incontinence: In extreme situations, rectal prolapse may cause fecal incontinence, or the involuntary passage of feces.

5. Pain or Discomfort: Women who have prolapse may feel pain or discomfort in their lower back, abdomen, or pelvic region. This discomfort may range in intensity from moderate to severe, and it could become worse with exercise or extended standing.

6. Sexual Difficulties: Prolapse may make it difficult or painful to engage in sexual

activity. Additionally, some females could express reduced sexual pleasure.

7. Lower Back discomfort: Uterine or vaginal vault prolapse may be accompanied by chronic lower back discomfort.

8. Vaginal Bleeding or Discharge: Vaginal bleeding or excessive discharge are sometimes caused by prolapse.

9. Difficulty Inserting and Retaining Tampons: Women with prolapse may have trouble inserting and retaining tampons.

It's crucial to remember that each person may have a different intensity level and set of symptoms. While some women may only feel a little pain, others may endure more severe symptoms that have a big impact on their quality of life.

You must see a doctor for a precise diagnosis and a customized treatment plan if you think you may have prolapse or are exhibiting any of these symptoms. Early diagnosis and treatment may lessen symptoms and stop additional prolapse-related consequences.

Prolapse diagnosis and medical evaluation

Prolapse is often diagnosed and evaluated medically by a doctor after a comprehensive examination. A medical history, physical examination, and maybe further testing or imaging investigations are all possible parts of the procedure. Here is a detailed explanation of the process for diagnosing prolapse:

Medical Background: A thorough medical history will be obtained by the healthcare professional first. They will inquire about your symptoms, including when they first appeared, how severe they were, and any circumstances that may have contributed to their occurrence. Your general health, past operations, pregnancies, and any other pertinent medical issues must all be disclosed.

Pelvic Examination: Diagnosing prolapse requires a thorough physical examination.

Your healthcare professional will examine your external genitalia during a pelvic exam to check for any obvious prolapse or abnormalities.

Assess the vaginal walls, cervix (if present), and vaginal vault using a speculum.

ask you to bear down or carry out certain movements to evaluate the kind and degree of prolapse. Observing the fall of pelvic organs such the bladder, uterus, or rectum may be necessary for this.

Pelvic Organ Prolapse Quantification (POP-Q) Assessment: The POP-Q system, a standardized technique for determining the degree of prolapse, is often used by healthcare professionals. It entails quantifying how much certain pelvic tissues have descended, and it offers a systematic method to evaluate and keep track of prolapse.

Assessment of Urinary and Bowel Function: Your doctor may ask you questions regarding your urination and bowel habits, including any incontinence problems, constipation, or problems emptying your bladder.

Imaging investigations (when needed): In certain circumstances, further examinations or imaging investigations may be needed to assess the prolapse's severity or to rule out other problems. These may consist of:

Ultrasound imaging of the pelvis may be used to assess the location and health of the pelvic organs and tissues.

Cystoscopy: This technique includes seeing within the bladder using a narrow tube equipped with a camera. It may aid in locating bladder-related problems brought on by prolapse.

Defecography: This specialist X-ray examination may shed light on bowel movement and rectal prolapse.

Evaluation of Related Symptoms: In order to make the best treatment decision, your healthcare professional may also assess any accompanying symptoms, such as urine incontinence or constipation.

Your healthcare professional will identify the kind and degree of the prolapse based on the results of these assessments and create a customized treatment strategy. Depending on your unique situation and preferences, treatment options may vary from dietary changes and pelvic floor exercises to the use of pessaries (vaginal devices) and surgical treatments.

It's crucial to keep lines of communication open with your healthcare practitioner throughout the diagnostic process since successful therapy and symptom alleviation of prolapse depend on an accurate diagnosis and appropriate evaluation.

Treatment Options

The types and degrees of prolapse, as well as specific patient variables and patient preferences, all influence the treatment choices for prolapse in women. Here is a summary of the many prolapse treatment options:

changes to one's way of life

Weight management: Keeping a healthy weight may lessen the stress on the muscles of the pelvic floor, lower the likelihood of prolapse, or ameliorate current symptoms.

Changing your diet may help avoid constipation, which can make the symptoms of prolapse worse.

Exercises for the Pelvic Floor (Kegel Exercises):

The pelvic floor muscles are contracted and then relaxed during kegel exercises. They could lessen discomfort by strengthening these muscles and enhancing pelvic organ support.

Physical therapy for the pelvic floor administered by a qualified therapist may provide advice on appropriate exercise methods.

Pessaries: In order to support prolapsed organs and treat symptoms, pessaries are vaginal devices that may be placed.

Depending on the nature and degree of the prolapse, several sizes and forms are available.

Prescription drugs may be used to treat certain prolapse symptoms like urine incontinence or an overactive bladder.

For postmenopausal women, hormone treatment, especially estrogen replacement therapy, may be explored to promote vaginal tissue health.

Surgical Interventions: Surgery may be advised if non-surgical therapies are ineffective or if the prolapse is severe. There are several surgical procedures available, such as:

Vaginal surgery: This might entail fixing the weakening tissue and giving the pelvic organs more support.

Abdominal surgery: In certain circumstances, this procedure is necessary since it may provide more thorough support and repair.

Hysterectomy: A hysterectomy, or removal of the uterus, may be advised in uterine prolapse instances. This procedure is often paired with other prolapse remedies.

Minimally Invasive Surgery: Compared to open surgery, laparoscopic or robotic-assisted procedures may result in faster healing periods and fewer incisions.

Surgical mesh has been used in the past to enhance repairs, but it has been linked to problems. Repairs without mesh are increasingly often requested.

Complementary treatments: Acupuncture, physical therapy, and biofeedback are examples of complementary treatments that some women use to treat the symptoms of prolapse.

Behavior modification and bowel training may be advised for those who have bowel-related symptoms in order to improve bowel habits and reduce straining.

Patient Education and Support: For women who are struggling with prolapse, education and support groups might be helpful. These sites provide knowledge, emotional support, and advice on symptom management.

The kind and degree of prolapse, general health, individual preferences, and the desire for future pregnancies should all be taken into consideration when deciding on a course of therapy. To explore the best course of therapy and develop a specialized treatment plan for your requirements, speak with a healthcare professional who specializes in pelvic floor diseases.

CHAPTER FOUR:

Prevention and Self-care

Preventing prolapse and taking care of oneself may help preserve pelvic floor health and lower the likelihood of prolapse symptoms appearing or becoming worse. Here are some self-care techniques and preventative measures:

1. Pelvic Floor Exercises (Kegel Exercises): Perform Kegel exercises often to build up the muscles in your pelvic floor. These exercises might strengthen the pelvic floor and lessen prolapse.

Consider seeking advice from a pelvic floor physical therapist since proper technique is crucial.

2. Maintain a Healthy Weight: By eating well and exercising regularly, one may achieve and maintain a healthy weight that puts less stress on the pelvic tissues and lowers the chance of prolapse.

3. Proper Lifting Techniques: When lifting big things, use the right body mechanics.

Keep your back straight, bend at the knees, and avoid doing heavy lifting whenever you can.

4. Prevent Constipation: Eat a diet rich in fiber to avoid constipation and uncomfortable bowel motions. Healthy bowel function also depends on enough water.

5. Control Chronic Cough: If you have a persistent cough, consult a doctor for care that will address the underlying issue. Pelvic floor tension might result from coughing.

6. Pelvic Support During Pregnancy: To alleviate some of the strain on your pelvic

floor when pregnant, think about using a belly band or pregnancy support garment.

7. Maintaining excellent Hygiene: To stop the transmission of germs and lower your risk of urinary tract infections (UTIs), maintain excellent hygiene by washing your hands from front to back after using the restroom.

8. Don't Lift hard Things While Pregnant: The extra weight of hard lifting during pregnancy might damage the pelvic floor. Use safe lifting procedures and seek help when necessary if you must lift anything large.

9. Avoid High-Impact workouts: Pelvic floor pain may result from high-impact workouts like jogging or leaping. Think about including lower-impact activities like cycling, walking, or swimming in your workout regimen.

10. Awareness of Pelvic Floor Health: Keep track of any physical changes and your pelvic floor's condition. Seek quick medical attention if you develop symptoms including pelvic pressure, pain, or changes in bowel or bladder function.

11. Regular Check-ups: - Arrange regular gynecological examinations so that you may

talk to your doctor about any issues relating to pelvic health.

12. Physical therapy for the pelvic floor: Consider speaking with a pelvic floor physical therapist if you exhibit prolapse risk factors or early warning signals. They may provide you individualized workouts and advice to support and develop your pelvic floor.

Always keep in mind that preventative measures and self-care techniques might change depending on the situation. It's essential to speak with a healthcare professional, particularly if you have certain risk factors or worries about prolapse. They can help you create a strategy to maintain pelvic floor health and provide you individualized advice and counseling that is catered to your requirements.

Effect on Life Quality:

A woman's quality of life may be significantly impacted by prolapse, which can have an influence on her physical, mental, and social wellbeing. The precise effect may change based on the prolapse's kind and degree as well as unique elements. The following are some typical ways that prolapse may reduce quality of life:

Physical pain and Pain: Prolapse often causes physical pain, such as pelvic pressure or heaviness. When doing tasks like standing, walking, or lifting, this pain may be ongoing or get severe.

Dyspareunia, which is discomfort experienced by some women during sexual activity, may also cause pelvic or lower back pain.

Bowel symptoms include constipation and diarrhea. Urinary symptoms include urinary incontinence (urine leakage), frequent urination, and a strong need to pee.

Fecal incontinence (involuntary bowel motions), constipation, and other gastrointestinal problems might also occur.

Sexual dysfunction: Women who have prolapse may feel pain or discomfort during sex, which may cause them to feel unsatisfied sexually and even put pressure on their relationships.

Impact on Emotions and Psychology: Prolapse may cause emotional discomfort, including feelings of humiliation, shame, or loss of self-esteem as a result of modifications in sexual or body image.

Coping with ongoing pain and lifestyle restrictions may lead to the development of anxiety and despair.

Impact on Daily Activities: Due to physical restrictions and pain, women with severe prolapse may find it difficult to participate in daily activities like exercise, work, or caring.

Social Isolation: Due to worries about incontinence or physical pain, some women may stop participating in social activities or avoid gatherings.

Limitations on Work and Productivity: Prolapse-related symptoms may have an impact on a person's ability to do their job, which may result in lost days of work or a decline in job satisfaction.

Impact on Family Planning: Women of childbearing age may need to think about how prolapse and possible treatments for it may influence their decisions about family planning and reproduction.

Financial Impact: Affected people and their families may experience financial hardship as a result of the expense of their treatment, which may include operations and drugs.

It's crucial to remember that each woman's experience with prolapse will be different, so not every woman will have all of these consequences. The kind of prolapse, how severe it is, whether or not there are any other medical disorders present, and the person's support network may all have an effect.

The quality of life for women who have prolapse may be greatly enhanced by seeking prompt medical examination and talking about treatment options with a healthcare practitioner. Effective care and support may lessen symptoms and deal with the mental and emotional difficulties brought on by this disease, enabling people to live more satisfying lives.

Prolapse may have a variety of psychological repercussions on women, typically as a result of the physical and emotional difficulties this disorder presents. Here are a some psychological side effects that prolapse sufferers often encounter:

Embarrassment and Shame: Women who have prolapse may experience feelings of embarrassment or shame while talking to others about it or seeking medical care. These emotions may be exacerbated by prolapse that is visible.

Loss of Self-Esteem: Prolapse-related changes in sexual function and body image may cause a person's self-esteem to drop. Women could feel less desirable or beautiful, which would affect their self-worth and self-confidence.

Anxiety and despair may result from coping with ongoing discomfort, suffering, and the uncertainty of having a prolapse. A sense of powerlessness and loneliness may make these mental health issues worse.

Sexual dysfunction: A decrease in sexual pleasure and desire may result from pain or discomfort experienced during sexual activity (dyspareunia). Intimate relationships and emotional health may be impacted by this.

Impact on romantic Relationships: The emotional toll of living with the illness and the sexual dysfunction caused by prolapse may strain romantic relationships, resulting in communication problems and diminished closeness.

Fear of Social Isolation: Women who worry about incontinence or pain may avoid social situations, which may result in feelings of loneliness and isolation.

Managing prolapse symptoms may be difficult, particularly if they interfere with routine tasks or obligations at work. For mental health to exist, appropriate coping strategies must be developed.

Impact on Family Planning: For women of childbearing age, prolapse may cause anxiety and emotional complexity by raising questions regarding family planning and reproductive options.

Financial worries: The expense of therapy, operations, drugs, and post-operative care may cause stress and worry.

Delay in Seeking Medical Care: Some women can put off getting medical help out of fear, shame, or a refusal to acknowledge their symptoms. This delay may make both psychological and physical impacts worse.

It's crucial to understand that psychological consequences might differ from person to person and may be influenced by the kind and degree of prolapse, unique coping mechanisms, and existing support networks. Integral treatment for those who have prolapse involves addressing the psychosocial effects of the condition. Therapy, support groups, and healthcare professionals may give emotional support, direction, and management techniques for these psychological impacts.

People with prolapse may be better able to manage their illness and enhance their general psychological wellbeing by seeking prompt medical examination, talking about treatment choices, and connecting with healthcare providers who specialize in pelvic floor issues.

CHAPTER FIVE

Recovery and Rehabilitation:

Medical therapy, self-care techniques, and lifestyle modifications are often used to promote prolapse recovery and rehabilitation. Depending on the nature and degree of the prolapse as well as the unique circumstances of each person, several approaches to rehabilitation may be necessary. Key components of healing and rehabilitation include:

A medical diagnosis:

The first stage of recovery is post-operative care if surgery was necessary to correct prolapse. This can include keeping an eye out for issues, controlling discomfort, and making sure surgical wounds heal properly.

Follow your doctor's recommendations for post-operative activity limitations, medication administration, and wound care.

Attend each and every post-operative visit as arranged to monitor recovery and resolve any issues.

Physical Therapy for the Pelvic Floor: Both before to and after surgery, physical therapy for the pelvic floor is often advised as a component of the recovery process. Guidance on pelvic floor exercises and methods to enhance muscular strength and coordination may be obtained from a qualified therapist.

To improve muscular function, the treatment strategy may combine electrical stimulation therapy and biofeedback.

Self-Care and Lifestyle Changes: Self-care is essential for both rehabilitation and continued prolapse treatment. Think about the following:

As advised by your doctor or physical therapist, keep up your pelvic floor exercises, such as Kegels.

By being active, eating a good food, and controlling your weight, you can keep up a healthy lifestyle.

Steer clear of strenuous activities that put pressure on the pelvic floor, such as heavy lifting.

Manage constipation by altering your diet and developing healthy bowel habits.

To avoid straining, drink enough of water and have frequent, healthy bowel motions.

To reduce urine and bowel discomfort, adopt healthy bladder and bowel practices.

Follow the insertion, removal, and maintenance guidelines provided by your healthcare practitioner if a pessary was recommended to support your pelvic organs.

To ensure appropriate installation and make any required modifications, attend routine follow-up consultations.

Support on an emotional level: For general wellbeing, it's crucial to address the prolapse's emotional effects. To discuss your thoughts and experiences, seek out help from friends, family, or support groups.

To assist handle any anxiety, despair, or emotional issues that may develop throughout recovery, think about seeking counseling or therapy.

Sexual Wellness:

Be upfront with your spouse about any modifications to your sexual function or comfort brought on by prolapse.

Talk with your healthcare practitioner about your choices if sexual dysfunction is a problem. These may include more counseling or treatment.

Continue scheduling routine follow-up visits with your doctor to address any lingering symptoms, check on your progress, and make any required modifications to your treatment plan.

Prolapse recovery and rehabilitation are often continuous procedures. Enhancing pelvic floor function, symptom relief, and general quality of life are the objectives. Together, you and your healthcare professional will create a customised strategy that caters to your unique requirements and guarantees the greatest result. It's crucial to heed their advice and keep lines of communication open throughout the healing process.

Prolapse patient experiences

Prolapse may have a broad range of effects on a patient's experience since each woman is affected by this ailment differently depending on the kind and degree of their prolapse, their coping methods, and the efficacy of their therapy. Here are some details of people's experiences dealing with prolapse:

Physical Symptoms and Discomfort: Many women with prolapse report experiencing bulging, heaviness, or persistent or sporadic pelvic pressure. These bodily signs may be uncomfortable and even unpleasant.

Daily challenges: Symptoms associated with prolapse might obstruct routine tasks. Long durations of standing or walking, exercising, and lifting large things may be challenging for women.

Impact on Intimate Relationships: Changes in some women's sexual comfort and function may make intimate relationships difficult. Intimacy may be impacted both physically and emotionally by these changes.

Emotional Impact: Coping with prolapse may be difficult on an emotional level. It's possible to have feelings of humiliation, shame, or poor self-esteem, especially when talking about your disease with others or getting medical help.

Coping strategies: To deal with prolapse-related symptoms and emotional difficulties, many people create their own coping strategies. These tactics could be asking loved ones for emotional support, participating in support groups, or looking into alternative treatments.

Treatment Experiences: Treatment outcomes might vary. While some women might find relief from conservative treatments like pessaries or pelvic floor exercises, others could need surgery to treat severe prolapse.

Impact on Family Planning: Women of childbearing age may have to make decisions about their reproductive and family planning options, which may complicate and emotionally tax their lives.

Support and Advocacy: Some women decide to promote prolapse support and awareness by sharing their own experiences and guiding others through the difficulties associated with the disease.

Resilience and flexibility: In managing their disease, many people with prolapse show resilience and flexibility. Despite the difficulties it poses, they manage to have happy lives.

Hope and healing:

Many women find that their symptoms and general quality of life improve with the appropriate care and encouragement. The road to recovery is often long, but there may be hope.

It's critical to understand that every woman's experience with prolapse is different. Others may find successful therapy and support networks that help them manage the disease effectively, although others may have substantial physical and mental issues.

For people who are struggling with prolapse, it might be crucial to seek help from loved ones, support groups, and medical professionals. Individuals may negotiate the physical and emotional components of this disease and strive toward greater well-being with the aid of supportive healthcare and emotional support.

PROLAPSE IS A MEDICAL CONDITION THAT HAS A SIGNIFICANT IMPACT ON THE LIVES OF MANY WOMEN IN THE WORLD. It includes the displacement or sinking of the pelvic organs, which causes pain on the physical, emotional, and societal levels. Women of all ages may have prolapse, which has a broad range of reasons and degrees of severity.

Distressing physical prolapse symptoms include pelvic pressure, bowel and urine issues, and discomfort. Furthermore, it is important to recognize the emotional costs of prolapse, such as feelings of humiliation, shame, and low self-esteem.

For women who are struggling with prolapse, there is, nevertheless, hope and assistance available. The quality of life for people afflicted may be considerably enhanced by early diagnosis, individualized treatment regimens, and successful coping techniques. Options for treatment vary from conservative ones like pessaries and pelvic floor exercises to surgical ones when required.

Additionally, educating people about prolapse and offering assistance via medical professionals, support networks, and loved ones may assist women in coping with the difficulties associated with this illness. Women who have dealt with prolapse may find inspiration and encouragement from their stories and tenacity.

In the end, it's important to remember that prolapse is a problem that can be treated, and there is a network of medical experts and patients waiting to give support, understanding, and optimism. Women may take proactive measures for improved pelvic health and a higher quality of life by treating

the psychological and physical components
of prolapse.